All You Need is Epsom Salt, Honey And Baking Soda

The Big Book Of Home Remedies For Health, Beauty, Cures, Natural Cleaning, Cooking, Crafts, Weight Loss And More

CECIL CROSS

ISBN-13:978-1535116008

ISBN-10:1535116005

DEDICATION

To my daughter, Annabel; watching you grow always make my day!

TABLE OF CONTENTS

INTRODUCTION

In a bid to lead a high quality of life, we spend lots of money on commercial beauty products, chemical cleaners, health supplements and medicines. But little do we know that there are some seemingly insignificant natural substances within our reach that could do so much more for us in a safer, healthier and inexpensive way.

Epsom salt, honey and baking soda, stored in our pantry will work wonders on our health, environment and home. Inside these items are many hidden natural beauty secrets, healing, cures, and home remedies that will address a staggering range of health issues, skin flaws, beauty needs, household needs, vegetation requirements, and interior décor. In fact, there are more than 200 ways to make use of these items to satisfy your desire for qualitative life!

What's more; there is no fear of endangering the health of your family and your pets with the high-priced toxic cosmetics and cleaners in the market. Epsom salt, honey and baking soda are all natural. They are also safe, affordable, non-toxic, environmentally friendly, incredibly versatile and 100 percent effective. By using them, you will lead a healthier life in a healthy home and environment.

This big book of three parts will open you to that world of possibilities. It will unravel secrets that may put commercial manufacturers and pharmaceuticals out of business.

So take a back seat and learn from the wealth of information contained therein. All you need is Epsom salt, Honey and Baking Soda!

PART I: Epsom Salt

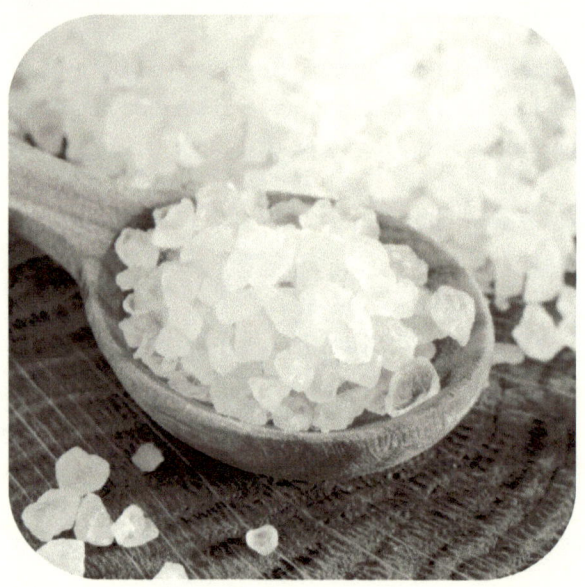

What Is Epsom Salt?

Epsom salt, also known as magnesium sulfate is a pure, natural occurring mineral compound with tremendous healing and beautifying properties. It is named after a bitter saline spring located in Epsom in Surrey, England. Its discovery was in 1618, after a farmer noticed that while his cows were unhappy with the bitter taste of the spring water from which they drunk, they were healed of their scratches and rashes. The good news of Epsom salts soon spread far and wide as more and more people attest of its efficacy. Today, Epsom salt is obtained generally from mining operations. They come in crystal forms, are inexpensive and can be purchased easily online or at drugstores in bags or boxes.

What Does It Do?

Epsom Salt should not be mistaken for table salt; they are not the same substance. Table salt is simply sodium chloride. It has no beneficial properties that can relieve the body, soul and mind. Epsom Salt, on the other hand, is made of two vital components - magnesium and sulfate; a mineral combination known for its therapeutic properties. It is a long-time remedy that has been proven to address a wide range of health issues such as curing skin troubles, treating cold and congestion, relieving body pains and aching limbs. It also helps to relax the nervous system and muscle strain, heal cuts, reduce soreness from childbirth and detoxify the body. As a matter of fact, you have the natural solution to the aches and pains you experience daily, right there in your pantry!

Besides its ability to heal the body naturally from many common ailments and health conditions, Epsom salt also offers several beautifying, household and gardening-related benefits. For beauty purposes, it has the ability to beautify and purify the skin, making it look beautiful, youthful and soft. For household applications, Epsom salt is a very useful home remedy with numerous cleaning purposes. This is why manufacturers of beauty and cleaning products often use it as part of their ingredients to make commercial hair products, cleaners, pedicure solutions and so on. Nevertheless, it is better, safer and cheaper to reach out for your own Epsom salt than to depend on commercial products that also has artificial fragrances and harmful chemicals on their labels.

This very powerful inorganic salt is a great garden supplement as well; helping to create healthy vibrant greenery, full roses and lush grass as well increasing the flavor of fruit and vegetables and plants nutrient uptake. Epsom salt is a natural fertilizer; enhancing the soil's capabilities to generate upmost vitality, to your garden's composition. You can also have fun with Epsom salt; creating paintings, cards, decorative bath crystals, vases, campaign bottles, glasses or shimmer candles with children. You can also decide to frost your windows for the season or create just about anything beautifully glimmering and shiny to celebrate Christmas, Halloween, Easter, Valentine or the Holidays.

Epsom Salt Facts You Should Know

Like any other product, Epsom salt can be dangerous if taken incorrectly. For instance, it should never be ingested without prior consultation with your doctor. It should also be taken in the right amount and frequency. Pregnant women and those with health concerns are also advised to check with their doctor before using.

Nevertheless, Epsom salt is a very dependable supplement that is generally applied topically or by soaking. The magnesium and sulfur it contains break away when immersed in liquid and are absorbed through the skin.

Magnesium plays major roles in the body. One of its functions is to regulate the activity of more than 320 enzymes. Magnesium helps to produce adenosine triphosphate (ATP), the energy packets made in the cells while the produced ATP helps to increases energy and stamina. This is why bathing with Epsom salt is often recommended by experts to gain more energy and generally feel better.

 Other functions of magnesium include helping to lower blood pressure, improving sleep and concentration, reducing inflammation, helping the nerves and muscles to work excellently and making insulin more effective. When your raise your magnesium levels through regular Epsom salt applications, you will enjoy several health benefits. Epsom salt makes insulin works better, and this helps to lower the severity or risk of diabetes.

The body loses magnesium when it is stressed, but Epsom Salt is a natural stress reliever. Once the body is soaked in a bath of Epsom salt dissolved in warm water, the skin absorbs Magnesium Sulfate and replenishes the level of magnesium the body needs.

The sulfates in Epsom salt help to flush toxins from the body and make it easier for nutrients to be absorbed into the body. It also helps to alleviate migraine headaches.

Epsom Salt's Sulfur And Detoxification

Successful detoxification of waste and toxins from the body can be achieved only when there is enough sulfur to do the work. Low levels of sulfur can cause toxin buildup which could affect our central nervous system. While there are other sulfur supplements available, most of them cannot penetrate the body with ease, and therefore, cannot provide the required effect. Epsom salts however, provides sulfates in a form that can readily be absorbed into the body. The provided sulfates make toxins and waste products water soluble, and consequently, they are excreted easily.

USES OF EPSOM SALTS FOR IMPROVED HEALTH

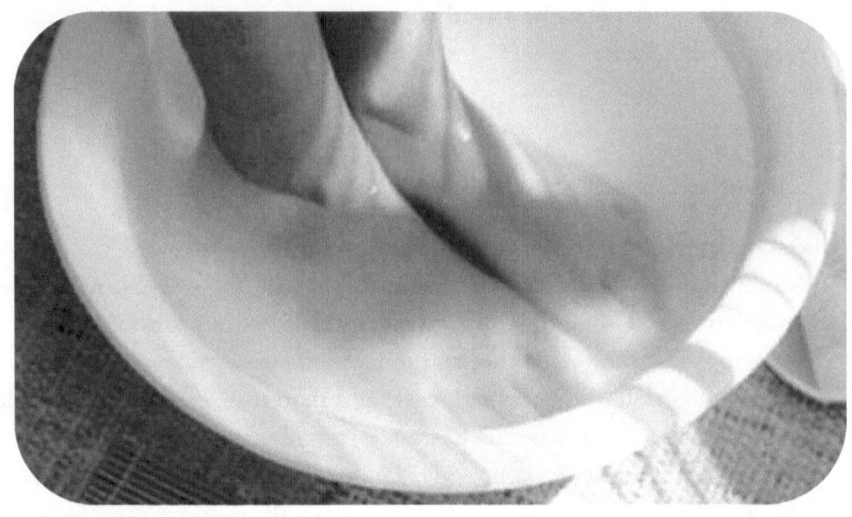

For Cramps, Aches And Pains

<u>Ease Muscle Pain</u>

1. Add 2 cups of Epsom Salt to warm water in a regular-sized bathtub. (Double amount of Epsom salt for oversized garden tub).

2. Soak for about 15 minutes. Have this bathe three times in a week.

<u>Menstrual Cramps Soak</u>

Simply toss 1-2 cups Epsom salts into the bath and soak away.

<u>Reduce Achy Bum</u>

If you have been riding in your bike all day in the country and your bum is sore and achy. Epsom salt will help. Just add 2 cups to a warm bath and soak your body.

<u>Epsom Salt Glow</u>

To help frequent headaches, provide relief from stiffness and arthritis as well as to improve skin condition.

1. Add1-2 cups Epsom salts to a container.

2. Add a few drops of water to it. The mixture will have a wet sand consistency.

3. Take mixture by handfuls and briskly rub over skin, avoiding the eyes until the entire body is done.

4. Rinse off in the shower and towel dry.

5. Do this regularly to help frequent headaches, to provide relief from stiffness and arthritis as well as to improve skin condition.

Heart Heath Improvement

Epsom salts improves blood circulation thereby preventing heart disease and strokes. It also prevents blood clots, protects the elasticity of arteries and reduces the risk of sudden deaths caused by heart attacks. Apply the Epsom Salt Glow treatment.

For Injuries

<u>Stubborn Splinters</u>

Combine ½ cup Epsom salt with 1 cup very hot water (the hotness of the water depends on what you can bear). Soak the splintered foot in the water, stirring around the salt to dissolve and soak until the waters begins to cool. Pat the area dry.

<u>Soothe Sprains And Bruises</u>

Sprains and bruises can be painful. Reduce this pain by adding 2 cups of Epsom salt to a hot bath and then soaking in the affected area.

<u>Epsom Salt Compress</u>

This can be used for bug bites, splinter removal and sore muscles.

Add 2 cups of Epsom Salt per 1 gallon of water for the compress.

<u>Reduce Inflammation</u>

Add 2 to 3 teaspoons of Epsom salts to a basin of very hot water and immerse the affected foot/joint. Soak feet for 20- 30 minutes.

For Skin Troubles

Bug Bite Itch

Add 1 teaspoon of Epsom salt to 1/4 cup of hot water, dissolve and let it cool. Dip a cotton ball or a piece of cloth in the solution, dab on the affected bite areas and be relieved of your itch.

Burns Treatment

This is an unbelievably effective treatment. What you need to do is to keep a jar of Epsom salts solution in your medicine cupboard or refrigerator as you never know when an accident in form of a burn can occur. When it does, simply pour the solution in a bandage or cloth on the affected area immediately. If the burn occurs on your fingers, just dip them into the jar for a couple of minutes.

For deeper burns, wash a raw potato and blend; mix the blended potato with Epsom salts and then apply as a cold poultice. Repeat this treatment on a regular basis until healed.

Aches & Itches Bath Salt Recipe

1 cup Epsom salt

1/2 cup baking soda

1 cup sea salt

1/2 cup dry milk

Directions

Combine all the ingredients in a large ziploc bag. Use in the bath as needed.

As Treatment For The Feet

With Epsom salts, you can lessen swelling in your foot, soothe inflammation and draw out infection.

Athlete's Foot

Dissolve Epsom salt in water and soak your feet in the solution for a few minutes. This will help relieve the symptoms of Athlete's Foot.

Ingrown Toenail Soak

Add about 1/2 cup Epsom salt per gallon of warm water and then soak the affected foot 15 to 20minutes. Do this procedure three times a day. This helps to soften the nail and makes it easier to trim.

Ease Gout Discomfort

Add 2 to 3 teaspoons of Epsom salts to a basin of very hot water and immerse the affected foot/joint. Soak feet for 20- 30 minutes.

Soothe Tired, Achy Feet

Refresh your feet

Add 1/2 cup of Epsom salt to a large bowl of warm. Add 1-2 drops peppermint oil as well. Soak your feet for 15-30 minutes.

Treat Toenail Fungus

Soak affected toes in hot water mixed with 1 cup Epsom salt. Do this three times in a day.

Eye Washes For Conjunctivitis, Cataracts, Irritation And Sties

Make a solution of Epsom salt and warm water and bathe the eye while it is closed. Do this thrice a day or as needed. If Epsom salt comes in direct contact with your eye, flush eye with water. If irritation persists, seek medical attention

Salt Drench For Insomnia, High Blood Pressure And Bedwetting

The salt drench method is highly effective because of the concentrated solution that is left on the skin. It is a very valuable aid in insomnia due to its powerfully relaxing effect. Regular use of this treatment can lower high blood pressure and help children with bed wetting. Desired results can become noticeable at least a week after continued treatments.

What To Do

1. Dissolve 2 oz. of Epsom salt in 1 a quart of warm water.

2. Take a hot bath or shower to help open pores. Do this every evening.

3. After the shower or bath, pour the solution slowly over your whole body and as far as you can, to cover each part.

4. Let it stay on your body for 1-2 minutes then pat dry body with a towel. Do not rinse it off. However, the waiting time before pat- drying depends on each individual. Some people will discover that they feel so relaxed, their limbs are heavy they find it hard to move. Experiment with waiting time and how thoroughly to dry to obtain a good night sleep and awake refreshed in the morning.

5. If you have a bedwetting child, bath the child and pour on the solution on him or her, wait a while and pat dry. This remedy can also be used for high blood pressure.

6. A simpler method to beat insomnia and improve sleep time is to just add 1 cup of Epsom salt to your bath of water. This will help you sleep.

Epsom Salt For Constipation

Epsom salt has been proven to be an effective home treatment for constipation. Its effectiveness is due to two main factors:

1. Epsom salt draws water from its surroundings; this softens stools and makes it easier to pass.

2. The magnesium contained in Epsom salt helps the bowel muscles to contract, making passing easier.

<u>What To Do</u>

Add 2 teaspoons of Epsom salt to 1 cup water or your favorite fruit juice and stir to dissolve. For children use ½ teaspoon of salt. Drink all in one sitting. There should be signs of bowel movement within 6 hours. If there isn't any sign, take one more dose. Do not forget to use only ½ teaspoon of Epsom salt for children. However, it is advisable to consult your physician before taken Epsom salts orally.

Boost Your Magnesium Level With Epsom Salts

If you are magnesium deficient but hate taking vitamins. Epsom salt can help. Simply dissolve in bath water and take a bath. The mineral is absorbed into your body easily. You have the required level of magnesium done safely and without ingestion.

However, if you want to take it internally, simply dissolve in a glass of water. As an adult, do not take more than 6 teaspoons per day. As a matter of fact, the recommended dose for adults is 2-6 teaspoon while children are 1-2 teaspoon. Be sure to use pure Epsom salts as well, without any added colorings or scents. Be warned though, it tastes horrible and poses some health risk if overdosed on! Then again, you may choose to take them in pill form if you really want to boost your magnesium level internally.

USES OF EPSOM SALT FOR BEAUTY

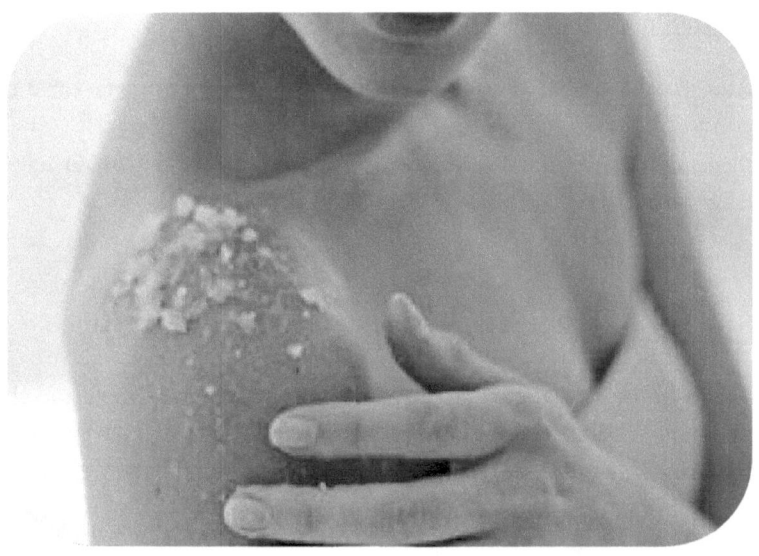

For Exfoliation

To exfoliate dead skin and soften it, wet your skin in the shower or bath and then mix a handful of Epsom salt with 1 tablespoon of olive oil. Rub mixture all over your body and then rinse well.

To clean your face, mix ½ teaspoon of Epsom salt with your favorite cleansing cream. Massage gently into skin and rinse face with cold water.

To Fight Blackheads

Add 1teaspoon Epsom salt and 3 drops of iodine into a ½ cup of boiling water. Dip a cotton ball in this mixture and apply to the blackheads.

For Your Hair

Create Pretty Hair Waves For The Beach

Add ½ tablespoons Epsom salts, 1/4 teaspoon of your favorite hair conditioner and 1 cup of hot water in a bottle with a nozzle. Shake thoroughly and then spray on damp hair. Crumble with your hands and leave to air dry.

Hair Volumizer

Add together equal parts Epsom salt and deep conditioner and then warm in a pan. Work this warm mixture through your hair. Leave it on for 20-30 minutes. Rinse thoroughly.

Remove Hairspray

Combine 1 cup Epsom salt, 1 gallon of water and 1 cup of lemon juice. Cover mixture and set aside for 24 hours. Pour this mixture into your dry the next day and leave it on for at least 20 minutes. Shampoo hair as normal.

Remove Excess Oil From Hair

Combine 9 tablespoons of Epsom salt and 1/2 cup of any oily hair shampoo. Apply 1 tablespoon of the liquid combination to your hair when dry and rinse hair with cold water. Next, Pour organic apple cider vinegar or lemon juice through the hair. Let it stay for 5-10 minutes and then rinse.

Chapped Lips Removal

Reduce those flaky skins hanging off your lips with some Epsom salt and petroleum jelly. Simply combine a dash of Epsom salt and some petroleum jelly. Rub on your palms and apply gently on your lips, wipe it off. The loose dead skin will reduce with constant application.

Eliminate Foot Odor/ Calluses

To remove bad foot odor, mix a ½ cup Epsom salt in warm water and soak feet for 10- 20 minutes. Use a pumice stone to rub calluses away and then dry feet. If you like, you can add 2 drops peppermint essential oil to a natural moisturizer like coconut or Shea butter.

Skin Renewals & Baths With Epsom Salt

Mix a small handful of Epsom salt with 1 tablespoon of olive oil and a drop of essential oil, rub all over your wet skin and then rinse well. Find below salt bath recipes to renew the skin, making it youthful, soft and smooth. However, if you have eczema or any preexisting skin condition, you may want to add essential oil or carrier oil like olive oil to your bath water. This will help to prevent further skin irritation that might result, leaving you to enjoy the therapeutic benefits of an Epsom Salt bath.

Home-Made Bath Glows

Ingredients

1 cup Epsom salt

1/2 cup Grape seed oil

1/4 cup Avocado oil

1 tsp. Vitamin E oil

20-30 drops essential oil blend

Directions

1. Combine bath salts and then set aside.

2. Combine oils and pour into an airtight jar.

3. Pour the bath salts into the jar and mix thoroughly. Store in a cool dark place

Cleansing Fragrant Salt Glow

Ingredients:

1/4 cup of Epsom salts

1/4 cup of sea salt

1/4 cup almond oil

1 tbsp borax

1 tbsp baking soda

4 drops lavender essential oil

8 drops geranium essential oil

Directions

1. Combine the salts in a jar, mixing well. Add borax, then baking soda and mix again.

2. Add essential oils and almond oil together then mix with the salts mixture. Now add the oils to the mixture. Mix well and store.

Pyramid Nights

Ingredients:

1/4 cup of Epsom salt

1/2 cup organic sea salt, crushed

3 drops Egyptian musk fragrance oil

Directions:

Combine ingredients, mix well and store in an air tight jar for up to 6 months.

Ocean Blue Bath Salt Recipe

Ingredients

1 cup of Epsom salt

1 cup baking soda

3 drops Jasmine fragrant or essential oil

4 drops blue food coloring

2 tablespoons glycerin

4 drops vanilla

Directions

1. Combine the dry ingredients, mixing well.

2. Add scents and color one at a time while stirring continuously until well mixed.

3. Break up clumps, if any. Continue to mix until a semi fine powder is attached.

4. Now add the glycerin and mix well.

Soothing Oatmeal Bath Salt Recipe

Ingredients

3 cups Epsom salt

1.5 cups finely pulverized oatmeal

10 drops lavender essential oil

Preparation:

1. Grind oatmeal finely in a food processor.

2. Mix the salts together. Add blended oatmeal to salts.

3. Add the essential oil and mix thoroughly. scoop mixture into airtight jars

4. Add the salt- oatmeal to running water and have a soothing soak. enjoy!

Epsom Salt, Detox And Weight Loss

Detoxification is the process of eliminating toxins and poisons from your body through the pores in your skin. Having regular detox bath at least 3 times a week will eliminate toxins from your skin and help you lose weight. They should be done in the evenings because you may feel tired or experience flu symptoms afterwards.

Start with 1 tablespoon of Epsom salt added to your bath water. You can increase the amount of Epsom salt gradually until you attain a maximum of 2 cups. This is because starting off with 2 cups may lead to hyperactivity, irritability and mood swings. Also, you may add vinegar or baking soda to get maximum benefit from the bath.

Kindly note that detox baths with Epsom salt is not advisable for people with high blood pressure, diabetes and heart trouble. It is safer and more effective to apply the salt glow method or salt drench method discussed in the preceding chapter.

Epsom Salt Detox /Weight Loss Baths

Ginger

Ginger will help your pores open up, making you to sweat a lot and eliminating toxins in the process. Add together 2 cups Epsom salt and 2 tablespoons grated ginger. Add combination in very hot water (as long as you can bear it) and soak body in for about 30 minutes.

Baking Soda

If using baking soda, simply add 2 cups of each in the bath water and rub body gently with a soft sponge.

Apple Cider Vinegar

For apple cider vinegar, use with Epsom salt in a ratio of 2:1. Add to warm water and soak for 40 minutes.

HOUSEHOLD USES OF EPSOM SALT

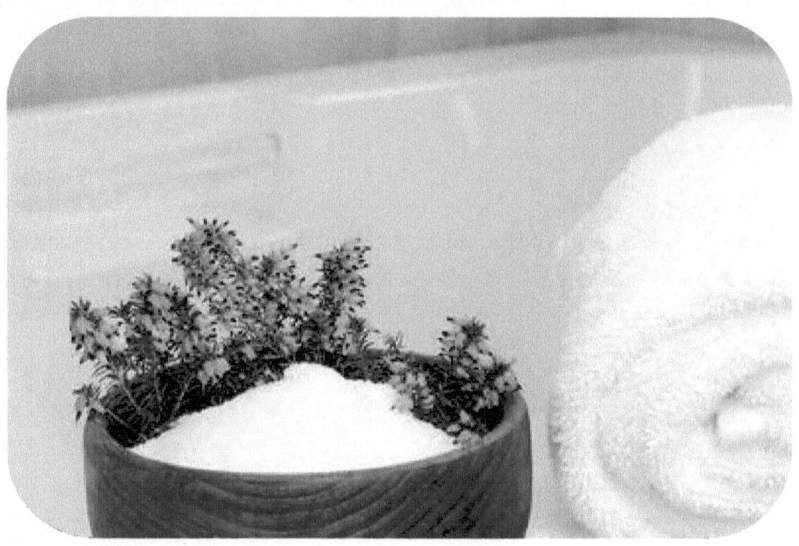

Bathroom Tile Scrub
Combine equal parts Epsom salt and liquid dish detergent and use mixture to scrub your bathroom tiles.

Remove Burnt Food Removal
Wash pans and pots with 1/4 tablespoon of Epsom salt and warm water and then rinse.

Hand Wash
For an effective hand wash, combine Epsom salt with any baby oil and keep by the kitchen sink.

Remove Detergent Build-Up On Your Washing Machines

Detergents often accumulate on washing machines. To clean them up, fill the tub with very hot water, add some Epsom salt. Run the machine. Let it agitate then soak and agitate again. This should dissolve the build-up of detergents in it. You may want to also consult your washing machine's instructional manual for detailed instructions.

Regenerate A Car Battery

Add together 1ounce warm water and Epsom salt to make a paste. Add paste to battery cells and give it more life.

Frost Your Windows For The Holidays

Epsom salts can help add some festive cheer to your home. Simply combine 1 cup Epsom salt, 3 tablespoon of dish soap and ½ cup boiling water. Dab onto your windows with a clean sponge. Once the mixture dries, your windows will wear a frosty look. Thanks to Epsom salt.

No- More Pesky Raccoons

Sprinkle some Epsom salt around the trash and drive those pesky raccoons away. This can help at campgrounds as well. Add more salts when it rains so the salts don't get all washed away.

USES OF EPSOM SALT IN YOUR GARDEN

Epsom salts help to facilitate the growth of your plant and increase the flavor of fruit and vegetables. They also help to increase plants nutrient uptake, deter pests and increase the production of vegetation. Simply sprinkle Epsom salt once in a week on your houseplants, flowers and vegetables to help nourish them. Before applying nutrients to soil however, it is always better to do a soil test.

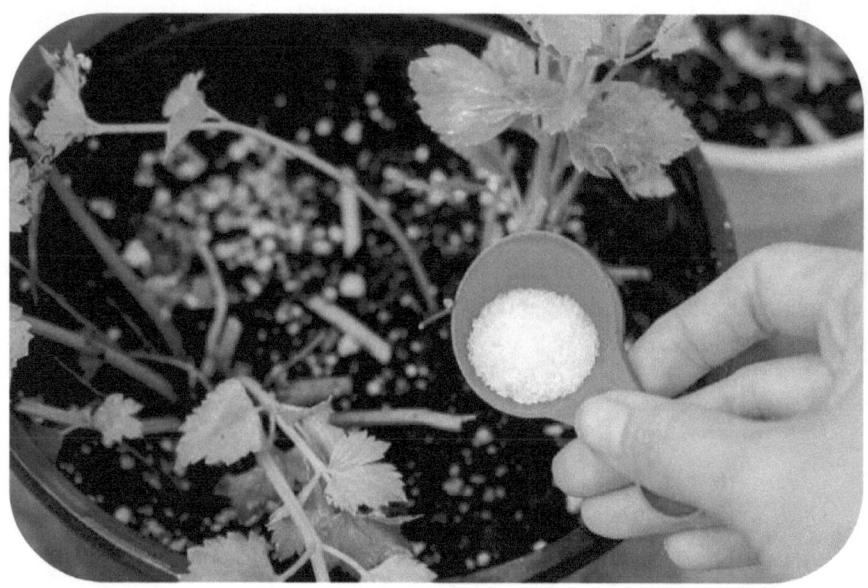

General Planting

Pre-Planting Soak

Before planting, dilute 1/2 cup of Epsom salt in 1 gallon of water and then soak the root balls in the solution.

Starting Your Plants

Dig hole for the planting, but before you plant seedlings or new plants, add I tablespoon of Epsom salt in the bottom of the dug hole. Cover this hole thinly with dirt and then place the plant in the hole.

Top Dressing

During the growing season, sprinkle 1 tablespoon of Epsom salt directly around the base of the plant and then water it in.

Drenching

Drenching plants with Epsom salt provides the plants with the required magnesium and consequently improves the general health of the plant. If your plants require a dose of magnesium, simply dissolve 1-2 tablespoons Epsom salt in1 gallon of water. Pour the solution at the base of the plant and let it soak into the ground. Repeat as necessary throughout the season.

As Natural Fertilizers

Epsom Salt works as a natural fertilizer for gardens due to two major components, the magnesium and sulfur it contains. Magnesium is important for seed germination. It also facilitates the production of chlorophyll, the pigment in plants that is used to transform sunlight into food. It facilitates the absorption of nitrogen and phosphorus, two essential fertilizer components.

Sulfur contributes to chlorophyll production. Most fertilizers contain phosphorus, potassium and nitrogen. Sulfur makes these three nutrients work at their best.

Lawn Fertilizer- Dilute 3 pounds of Epsom Salt in water and spray on lawns. Apply for every 1,250 square feet with a spreader, or dilute in water and apply with a sprayer (use as a lawn fertilizer).

For Green Lawns

For healthy green grass, combine 2 tablespoons Epsom salt and 1 gallon of water. Sprinkle mixture on your lawn. This will prevent yellowing leaves and produce lush greenery.

Watering Can Method For Green Lawns

1 cup Epsom Salts

1 cup Household Ammonia

Mix ingredient together in a jar. Combine 2 tablespoon of this mixture and 2 gallons of water in a watering can. Sprinkle over 150 to 200 square feet of turf.

Hose Sprayer Method For Green Lawns:

Combine all the ingredients with enough water to make 1quart of liquid. Pour this liquid into a sprayer. This should cover about 2,500 square feet of lawn.

Tips:

Avoid a heavy dose of the solution in the middle of summer as this can stimulate weed. Do not apply to dry soil. Soil must be damp at all times when applying as natural fertilizer.

Weed Killer

Mix 2 cups Epsom salt with 1 gallon of vinegar. To this mixture, add liquid dish soap and pour into a spray bottle. Spray the weeds but be sure to avoid your flowers and other plants in the process. This should effectively kill the weeds without damaging your valuable plants.

Prevents Plant Pests

Get rid of crawling slimy slugs forever and prevent them as well. Sprinkle Epsom salt on interior entry point or near it. Epsom salt is non- toxic, so it is kid friendly.

Counter Transplant Shock

Transplant shocks occur when plant roots are damaged during relocation. Epsom salts help plants adapt to its new location by helping with chlorophyll production and improving nutrient uptake of fertilization.

Make your planting and then water these plants with a solution of1 tablespoon Epsom salt and 1 gallon of water.

Prevent Leaf Curling

Leaf curling in plants occurs when the plants do not have enough magnesium. Sprinkle Epsom salt to the soil and water it in or dissolve 1 tablespoon Epsom salt per gallon of water and drench soil thoroughly.

Tree Stump Removal

Epsom salt has the ability to absorb water from wood. This makes it easy to remove tree stumps. What you do to remove a tree stump is to drill plenty of holes, about three or four inches apart, in the top of the stump. Do this until there is no area left to be drilled. Now, pour Epsom salt into the holes and add water.

Exposed roots must also be dried. Pour Epsom salt onto them to dry out. If you are not successful the first time, repeat the process every 3 weeks until the stump decays and can then be removed without difficulty.

Epsom Salts For Your Roses

Epsom salts added to Rose plants make for darker green foliage, vibrant blooms and stronger plants. Applied regularly, Epsom salts will increase aid seed germination and the chlorophyll production process. It will make the cell walls stronger and increase the flow of nitrogen, sulfur and phosphorus to the plants.

During Planting –soak the roots of the Rose plants in 1/2 cup of Epsom salt diluted in 1 gallon of water. When planting the bush in the pot or ground, sprinkle 1 tablespoon of Epsom salt into the hole before you plant and cover thinly with a layer of soil.

Top Dressing – during the growing season, sprinkle 1 tablespoon per 1 foot of plant height Epsom salt around to the base of the plant and then water it in. do this once a month.

Healthy Tomatoes & Pepper

With Epsom salts added to your tomatoes and pepper plants, you can be sure of sweeter tomatoes, more blooms and more fruit, less blossom rot, increase yields, deeper green foliage and stronger plants.

<u>Sweet Tomatoes</u>

Combine 1 tablespoon Epsom salt and 1 a gallon of water and water the plants every two weeks. The solution absorbs into the plant easily and quickly. You may use warm water to help dissolve the salts faster.

<u>Planting Tomato And Pepper</u>

Follow the steps for General Planting above

Fruit Trees

Fruiting is a long process. During this season also, there is often a drop in the level of magnesium. Epsom salt can be of immense benefit by helping plants to grow stronger, improving photosynthesis and ultimately making the fruits to taste better, look more appealing, and be nutritious. They will also be resistant to climatic conditions and disease.

Apply 2 tablespoons of Epsom salt over the root zone for 9 square feet area. Do this three times in a year.

CLEVER USES OF EPSOM SALTS AS CRAFTS AROUND THE HOME

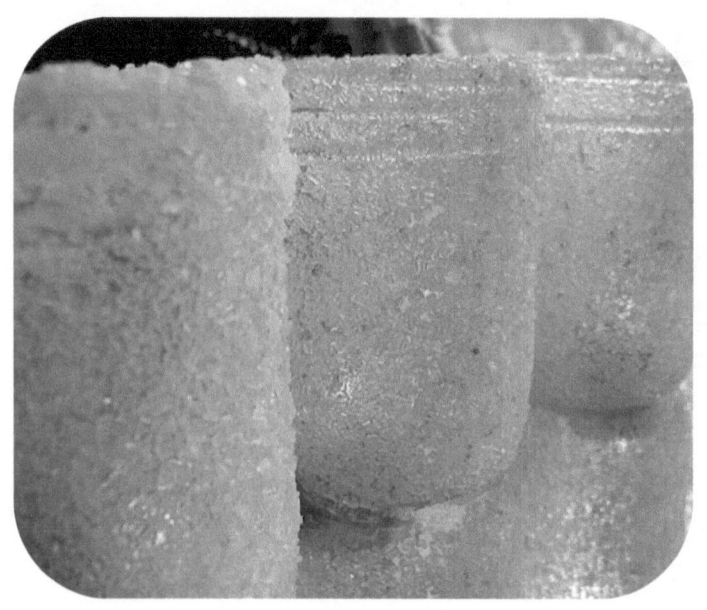

Epsom Salt Shimmery

Materials

1/4 cup Epsom salt

1/4 cup of hot tap water

Vases, jars, candle holders or bottles

Small bowl

Paper towel or rag

<u>Directions</u>

1. Wash glass well and dry. If glass is greasy the salt will not stick so wash thoroughly. Pour the hot water into the bowl and add the Epsom salt, stirring until dissolved. If necessary, microwave the solutions a few seconds.

2. Soak paper towel or rag in the salt solution and then wring out. Wipe the solution onto the glass and then leave to dry. (To get different looks, you may want to play around application styles by wiping horizontally, vertically or by dabbing, swirling and so on).

3. You may also apply plenty of layers while drying in between the layers, to make the glass appear opaque. However, you can change your results if you do not like the one you have done by washing the salt off with hot water and trying again.

Kids Snowy Scenes
<u>Materials</u>

Paper

Crayons

Brushes

Water

And of course Epsom salt

<u>Directions</u>

1. Have kids draw winter scenes and color them.

2. Combine 16 ounces of Epsom salts and 4 ounces of very hot water, stirring well to dissolve.

3. Have kids paint over the colored pictures with the mixture.

4. Frosty crystals will appear as the pictures dries.

Glimmer Paints

Make glossy, puffy paints that sparkle when dry.

½ cup Epsom salt

½ cup water

½ cup all-purpose flour

Food coloring

Directions

1. Combine Epsom salt, flour and water, until mixture attains a pudding-like consistency.

2. Add food coloring until preferred shade is attained. Transfer the paint to a squeeze bottle or Ziploc bag with a funnel.

3. Leave paintings overnight to air-dry. Store the leftover paints in airtight containers and refrigerated for up to three days. Stir before using.

Romantic Glitter Candle

<u>Materials</u>

1/2 cup Epsom salt

Plain pillar candle

Decorative flower

Spray adhesive

Glue dots

Red food coloring

Paper plate

<u>Directions</u>

1. Pour some Epsom salt into a bowl and add 1 drop red food coloring. Stir salt to distribute evenly and then pour onto a paper plate.

2. Spray the bottom half of the pillar candle with spray adhesive.

3. Roll candle in the Epsom salt until well coated.

4. Attach decorative flower to the front of the pillar candle with a glue dot.

5. Do not forget to take out the flower before burning the candle

Display Wine Bottles

<u>Materials</u>

Epsom salt

3 wine bottles

Primer

Adhesive spray

<u>Directions</u>

 1. Spray a coat of primer on the wine bottles and leave to dry.

2. Spray bottles with spray adhesive.

3. Pour Epsom salt onto a surface and roll bottles in it.

4. Place bottles on a silver tray and spread some Epsom salt around it.

You may want to place some small decorative items around the bottles and tray.

Sparkly Eggs For Easter

<u>Materials</u>

Epsom Salt

Plastic eggs

Small Paint brush

Glue

<u>Directions</u>

Paint glue on egg, roll egg in the salt and leave to dry.

Epsom Salt & Beer Window Frosting

<u>Materials</u>

1 cup of beer

8 tablespoons Epsom salts

Tissues

Soft towel

<u>Directions</u>

1. Add the salt to the beer. Leave for 30 minutes so the salt can partially dissolve.

2. Apply mixture to the window in a circular motion using a paintbrush or cloth.

3. Use a tissue to dab window while still wet and pat any running mixture on the glass.

4. You have your beautiful frosted window when mixture dries.

Glitter Sand For Candles & Mason Jar

Add food coloring to your Epsom salt. Mix thoroughly with hands. Pour in decorative mason jars. Epsom salt appears as glittery snows. Add a candle if you want. You can also make glittery candles by rolling them in Epsom salt.

Epsom Salt Snowman Vase

<u>Materials</u>

Epsom salt

Fish bowl vase

Decoupage or white, translucent glass paint

Small buttons or decorative brads (trim off tabs from the back)

Spray acrylic or lacquer sealer

Scissors

Ribbon

Foam brush

Hot glue

<u>Directions</u>

1. Apply a generous amount of paint on the outside of the vase. The vase should be well coated.

2. Sprinkle Epsom salts over the paint and leave to dry on vase. Once dry, shake off excess salt and then spray the vase with a clear sealer. The area must be well ventilated area. Apply many layers of sealant while allowing it to dry between layers. Wait for it to dry.

3. Meanwhile, cut the ends of the ribbon to create a scarf and then glue it onto the vase when it's dry. Add buttons or brads also.

4. There! You have your snow man.

PART II: Honey

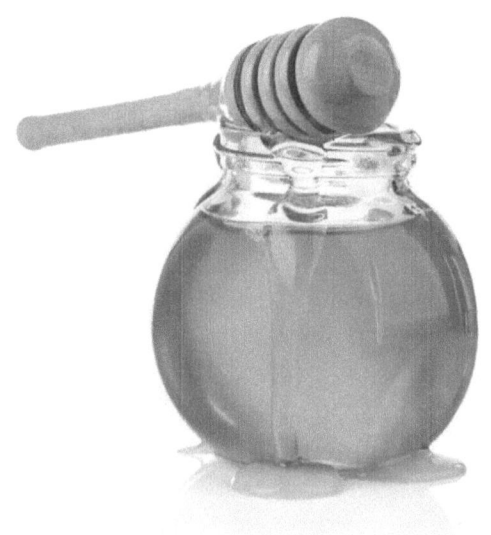

Honey—The Wonder Food

Honey is a pure and natural sweetener that has been consumed by man for centuries. Every year, the honey bees produce about 1 million tonnes of honey worldwide. Of this number, 285 million pounds are consumed by Americans alone.

Honey is a wonder food. It is one of the healthiest, most delicious and sustainable sweeteners in the world. It never seems to go bad, develop mold or contaminate even when it is not refrigerated after being opened. Archeologists reportedly found 2000-year old honey jars in Egyptian tombs and they were still fresh and tasted delicious!

Since bacteria love sugar, isn't it surprising that they cannot grow in honey? The reason is that honey is a natural antibiotic. It has a unique chemical composition of relatively high acidic level and low water content that creates a low pH environment, making it extremely unfavorable for bacteria to grow.

Think honey if you wish to enhance your health and that of your household. Its natural healing characteristic will help to control diabetics, cholesterol levels and blood sugar. This way, your body will heal faster than any supplements options in the market.

Honey has proven it can strengthen the immune system so it should be part of your daily diet (the darker, the better). It certainly makes sense to have a little raw honey every day because it will not only make you feel more energetic, but also help you to stay healthy.

However, do not give raw honey to children under the age of one as it contains the spores of botulinus. Infants who are of this age may not have the required stomach acid to stop these spores from developing. This may lead to botulism, a life-threatening disease.

Two Common Honey Varieties

While there are several honey varieties available, for the purpose of this book, we would consider Manuka and Raw honey, which are acclaimed for their extraordinary health benefits.

Manuka Honey

Made in New Zealand, Manuka honey is obtained from the nectar of Manuka flowers. Unlike other honeys, it contains an additional, naturally occurring active ingredient which is stable and sustains its potency even when it is exposed to light, heat or dilution. It has been clinically tested for wounds, herpes blister and skin ulcers treatments, It stimulates tissue healing.

Manuka honey can be used in treating many types of ulcers, post-surgical wounds, abscesses and fistulas. It is also used in treating non-healing wounds in cancer patients, as well as those induced by radiation therapy.

Raw Honey

Raw honey is the most original honey that the honeybees produce. It is honey that has not been heated or filtered. It contains small quantities of the same resins that are found in propolis. When extracted, the honey is warm and flows with ease. Consuming local raw honey provides you with immunization against allergies.

The Many Wonders Of Honey

It Is Nutritious.

Honey contains several vitamins like B6, riboflavin, niacin, thiamin, pantothenic acid and some amino acids and minerals such as copper, calcium, iron, magnesium, phosphorus, potassium, manganese, sodium and zinc.

It Is A Very Healthy Food Choice.

Honey's sugar absorb gently into the blood stream, resulting in better digestion.

It Energizes.

Honey is a natural carbohydrate source that provides the body with strength and energy. It helps to boost the performance and endurance of athletes.

Since it contains natural fruit sugars, glucose and fructose, it is able to prevent fatigue during exercises.

Additionally, honey contains no cholesterol thus including small quantities of it in the daily diet helps to keep the cholesterol levels in check.

It Builds Immunity Against Sicknesses And Diseases.

Honey contains antioxidants that help in eliminating free radicals and biologically harmful chemical agents that cause diseases like cancer.

It strengthens white blood cells and promotes blood formation. Honey also helps to supply the nutrient needed for the growth of new tissue.

It Beautifies You.

Honey has hygroscopic properties so it can be used as part of natural beauty recipes for skin care, hair care, facial scrubs, moisturizers and skin care.

It keeps the skin fresh and hydrated. With its natural anti-microbial and antioxidant properties, it rejuvenates and refreshes the skin, making it soft and supple.

It Acts As A Natural Remedy For Many Health Problems

Honey is the only natural sweetener that has healing effects. A wide range of health problems and ailments can be effectively treated with honey as you will soon discover in this book.

Medicinal Properties of Honey

Antibacterial

Antioxidant

Anti-allergic

Antiviral

Anti-inflammatory

Autoimmune protection

Eye health

Wound healing

Promotes calcium and selenium absorption

Prebiotic effect promoting healthy gut

Honey: Myth & Fact

<u>Fact</u>

- Honey is sweeter than table sugar
- Honey's quality or nutritional value is not affected by crystallization.
- Honey is a healthier option compared to artificial sweeteners.
- Honey contains zero cholesterol
- Honey helps your body to burn fat even while you are asleep

<u>Myth</u>

- Honey should never be scooped with a metal spoon — this is untrue. although honey is acidic; the action of scooping honey takes just a few seconds so corrosion cannot even occur.

- Honey is best mixed with hot water — this is untrue. Adding hot water to honey reduces its aroma and flavor and may also destroy a few healthy enzymes that are contained in it.

- Honey never spoils, even when stored in an open jar — this is untrue. If honey is left uncovered for an extended period of time, it will absorb moisture from the air and this will lead to fermentation.

- Honey can be bought in powder forms — this is untrue. Natural honey is only available in liquid forms and cream but not in powder form. Cactus honey powder should not be mistaken for natural honey as it is not produced by bees but from the juice of the agave cactus plant.

- Honey contains a little fat — this is untrue. Honey is 100% fat free

Cooking with Honey — Practical Tips

- Honey is nearly twice as sweet as sugar so use less of it when cooking.
  However, some honey varieties like Tupelo are sweeter than others.

- When cooking, replace 1 cup sugar for ½ cup honey. Honey also attracts water so reduce liquid quantity by 1/4 cup for every cup of honey added to the recipe.

- When baking, compared to sugar recipes, beat vigorously and for longer. Honey batter also becomes crisper and browns faster too. Simply lower the oven temperature by 25degree F.

- To neutralize the acidity of the honey, add 1/2 teaspoon of baking soda for each cup of honey. This will also help the food rise.

- When making use of honey in jellies, jams, or candies, raise the cooking temperature a little so that the extra liquid will evaporate.

- Honey has a way of enhancing, balancing, or imparting its flavor to other foods so consider its floral variety when cooking with it. The large number of mouthwatering recipes with honey that are available today is due to the many honey varieties and the versatile ways they are cooked.

Have these cooking qualities of honey at your fingertips:

- Extends shelf-life — a natural preservative for sauces and pickles.
- Enhances flavor — an excellent natural sweetener for cold beverages and hot teas.
- Provides feel and texture — a great addition in cake making and pastries.

- Adds color — contributes an agreeable golden hue to jellies, dressings, sauces and frozen desserts.
- Retains moisture — a vital ingredient that provides the moisture in quality cakes and prolong the moisture retention.
- Binding viscosity — a wonderful ingredient that helps the shaping of desserts like cakes, pastries and puddings.

Measuring Honey Accurately

Baking or cooking with a large quantity of honey can be messy and confusing. Learn how to get the precise measurement neatly and correctly.

1. Brush or smear the inside walls of a measuring cup with baking/cooking oil thinly and evenly all around it.

2. Pour the required amount of honey into the measuring cup.

3. The thin and even layer of oil makes it impossible for the honey to stick onto the cup.

4. You can now pour out the honey from the cup and none will be stuck to the measuring cup. Also, you do not need to scrap out the remaining honey from the measuring cup so as to obtain the accurate amount of honey as required in the recipe.

HONEY TREATMENTS FOR BEAUTIFUL SKIN

Honey treats blemishes effectively and helps the skin to retain its moisture. As a natural antiseptic, Honey is just right. It is the ideal ingredient for masks and cleansers. It will moisturize and condition your face, leaving no trace of oil.

Honey & Egg White Mask

1 tbsp honey

1 egg white

1-2 drops tea tree oil

Instructions:

1. Mix ingredients together. Apply on face and let it stay for 10-15 minutes.

2. Rinse face with warm water.

3. Refrigerate left over mask for up to 1 week

4. Use mask 2-3 times a week

Pore Refining Toner

1 tbsp honey

2 tbsp witch hazel

1 tsp lemon juice

Instructions:

1. Combine ingredients. Let it sit for 3-4 days before using. This way, the honey loses its stickiness.

2. Refrigerate toner.

Face Mask For Acne

Cinnamon exfoliates and will stimulate your pores. Nutmeg will even your skin tone and work as an anti-inflammatory as well. Lemon juice removes dead skin cells and aids fade scars.

3 tbsp honey

1 tsp cinnamon

1 tsp nutmeg

Lemon juice (optional)

Instructions:

1. Combine all ingredients in a small bowl until dark brown and slightly thick.

2. Refrigerate mixture to further thicken and make application easier.

3. Apply mixture to face, leave for 30 minutes, rinse and dry gently. Moisturize if needed.

4. Refrigerate the rest.

Rejuvenating Facial Mask

1 tbsp honey

1/4 cup dried apricots

1 tbsp dried milk

¼ cup water

Instructions:

1. Blend ingredients with electric blender.

2. Leave on face for 15 minutes. Rinse thoroughly.

Anti-Aging Skin Care Recipe

This recipe fights hydration. The honey will draw out skin impurities and moisturize naturally. This makes it the ideal ingredient for a homemade anti-aging skin care recipe.

1. Cleanse your skin. Apply 1tbsp honey all over the face.

2. Leave it for 10 minutes. Rinse off with warm water.

3. Add a tablespoon of brown sugar for extra exfoliating power

Honey Complexion Brightener

Equal part honey

Equal part Lemon juice

Instructions:

1. Mix together and apply to face and neck.

2. Leave it for 5-10 minutes then rinse.

Natural Skin Polisher

1tbsp sugar

11/2 cup honey

Instructions:

Mix together and use 2-3 times a week

HONEY TREATMENTS FOR HEALTHY HAIR

Honey contains potassium as well as vitamins A, B and C. These nutrients keep the hair healthy, moisturized, and shiny. Thus, it is the perfect treatment for conditioning hair. Use these honey hair treatments regularly as a preventative measure, for dry and brittle hair, to repair damaged hair as well as for color-treated hair.

Garlic – Honey Scalp Treatment

Garlic increases blood circulation to the scalp, helps to reduce hair loss and prevents dandruff. Honey protects the hair and makes it smooth and silky.

1/2 cup honey

Head of garlic

Shampoo Hair conditioner

Instructions:

1. Cut up cloves with cheese grater or mash in a garlic press.

2. Combine the honey and garlic in a bowl.

3. Using only your finger tips, rub this mixture into your scalp and hair. Do this for 5 minutes.

4. Rinse hair with warm water, wash with shampoo and then apply the conditioner.

5. Rinse with cold water to have a shiny hair.

Anti-Hair Loss

When it comes to treating hair loss, honey is a dependable natural ingredient. It will make your hair follicles really stronger.

1. Massage 1 tsp honey into your scalp. Let it stay for 1 hour then rinse off.

2. It can also be mixed with hair shampoo or conditioner.

Hair Strengthener

1 tbsp honey

½ cup olive oil

Instructions:

Mix and apply to the hair. Let it stay for 30-45 minutes then rinse off.

For Brittle Hair (caused by dry weather conditions)

1 tbsp honey

1 egg yolk

1 tsp olive oil

Instructions:

1. Mix together to make a rich hair conditioner

2. Use 1-2 times weekly

Hair Mask

Restore color, body and shine to your hair

1. Apply1/4 to 1/2 cup pure honey onto hair and wrap hair in plastic.

2. Leave honey-saturated hair on for 25 minutes. Rinse off

Hair Removal Wax

To remove hair effectively, honey wax must be kept at the right temperature. If it is too cold, it will create a difficult and sticky mess on your skin. If it is too hot, it could cause skin irritation or burns.

1 cup honey

1 cup white sugar

Juice of ½lemon

Instructions:

1. Combine sugar and honey in a small electric pot. Add lemon juice.

2. Set electric pot to low temperature, cover and cook for 2 hours. The honey should be thin and the mixture should be easy to stir using a flat wooden stick.

3. Leaving the electric cooking pot still on, remove lid for about 10 minutes for wax to cool for a while before you begin waxing.

4. Using a flat wooden stick, scoop up some wax and carefully touch it with your finger tip to ensure it is cool enough to use.

5. In a 4-inch long by 2-inch wide strip, spread the wax onto the desired skin area.

6. Next, press a strip of cotton fabric that is larger than the wax strip onto the warm honey wax. Smooth down the cotton strip by using your hands to rub it firmly 3-4 times.

7. Hold the skin around the strip firmly with one hand. Using the other hand to grasp the edge of the cotton strip, pull it off quickly in the opposite direction of the hair growth.

8. (Your hand should be very close to the skin when pulling off the strip so you wouldn't cause yourself unnecessary pain).

9. Keep applying and removing the wax the unwanted hair has been completely eliminated then gently wash the skin with warm water to remove any leftover wax.

10. Do not use lotions or soap as they may irritate your newly-waxed skin.

Honey Hair Rinse

For healthy and shiny hair

1tsp honey

4 cups very warm water

Instructions:

1. Combine ingredients and transfer to a plastic squeeze bottle.

2. Shampoo the hair and then apply this treatment to the scalp and hair.

3. Let it stay on for 2-3 minutes then rinse with warm water.

4. For best results, let the hair air dry. Use daily.

Honey Banana Deep Conditioner

This powerful solution coats the hair cuticles, resulting in locks that are healthy and manageable.

1 ripe banana, mashed

1tbsp pure honey

Instructions

1. Combine ingredients until a smooth consistency is achieved.

2. Next, dampen the hair with warm water. Take the mixture and massage it onto the hair and into the scalp.

3. Cover the hair with a clean towel, shower cap or plastic wrap and leave for 20 minutes before rinsing.

4. Shampoo and condition for the hair to air dry. Use it at least twice a week.

Honey Olive Deep Conditioner

3tbsp honey

1tbsp olive oil

Instructions:

1. Mix together until smooth. Shampoo hair and apply the mixture to it.

2. Let it stay for 15 minutes. Use warm water to rinse.

3. Apply once in a week. For very long hair, double the ingredients.

HONEY FOR MEDICINAL PURPOSES

Keep your body hydrated once you have a cold so that the congestion caused by the virus will be loosened with no difficulty.

COUGH SYRUPS

Honey-Lemon Cough Syrup

This very common homemade cough honey recipe is easy to make and highly effective for soothing sore throats and mild coughs.

16 ounces raw honey

1 lemon

Instructions:

1. Place the honey in a pan then cook on low heat but do not let it boil.

2. Bring a separate pan of boiling water to a boil, place lemon in it and leave to boil until the outer skin becomes soft. Leave to cool. Slice the softened lemon into 4 pieces.

3. Place the sliced lemon into honey and simmer on low heat for 1 hour. Pass mixture through a strainer to remove seeds and lemon. Let the mixture cool.

4. Once cool, place in a container, cover and put in the refrigerator for up to 2 months.

5. Take 4 times daily or as needed. Adults-1Tablespoon; children 50 pounds and above-1 teaspoon; and children under 50 pounds - ½ tablespoon.

Anise-Honey Cough Syrup

Anise helps to treat coughs, asthma and bronchitis.

2 cups honey

1 tsp anise seed, crushed

Instructions:

1. Bring 1½ cups water to a boil, place the crushed anise seed inside, cover and set aside for 30 minutes.

2. Pass liquid through a strainer, simmer until 1 cup remains then add honey and mix thoroughly.

3. Place in a sealed container and refrigerate. (Can last up to 2 months)

Horehound-Honey Cough Syrup

Horehound contains a phlegm-loosening expectorant. It is extremely effective in the treatment of coughs and colds.

Honey

1 ounce horehound leaves, dried

Instruction

1. Bring 16 oz water to a boil then place the horehound leaves in it. Let it sit 10 minutes.

2. Strain to remove the leaves. Next, add one part of the mixture to two parts honey, shaking thoroughly.

3. Place in an airtight jar and refrigerate for two months. Take 4 times daily or a

Honey Gargle For Sore Throats

For quick relief

3 tbsp raw honey

1/2 tsp cinnamon powder

1 cup hot water

Instructions

1. Mix ingredients together.

2. Gargle with this mixture 4-5 times daily to soothe your sore throat.

Or:

2 tbsp honey

4 tbsp squeezed lemon juice

Pinch of salt

Instructions

1. Mix ingredients together.

2. Gargle with this mixture 4-5 times daily to soothe your sore throat.

Honey Cough Drops

Natural, sweet and very effective!

1 cup raw honey

1 tsp cinnamon powder – optional

Instructions:

1. Boil honey to 300 degrees F. Pour mixture into small candy molds or drop 1/2 tsp amounts onto parchment paper.

2. Leave to cool completely before removing from parchment paper or molds. Enjoy!

Natural Flu Shot

Taste sour but works like hell!

3 tbsp raw honey

Juice of 6 lemons

3 cups Pineapple Juice

1 clove of garlic

1/4 tsp cayenne powder

Instructions:

1. Blend all the ingredients and store in a jar.

2. Take 1 cup four times daily until all symptoms disappear

Garlic& Honey Cold Treatment

Garlic and honey are natural antibacterial ingredients that fight cold-causing germs and boost the immune system.

½ cup raw honey

4 garlic cloves, peeled & sliced into 8 pieces

Juice of 1 lemon

Instructions:

1. Place garlic pieces in a saucepan, add 4 cups distilled water to it and bring to a boil on medium-high heat. Once mixture emits a garlic scent, remove from heat.

2. Add honey to garlic water, stir and add lemon juice to the mixture.

Arthritis Honey Remedy

Lemon helps to lessen the inflammation that causes arthritis.

1tsp honey

1 cup warm water

1-2 tsp lemon

Instructions:

Mix well and drink 5-6 times daily

Bad Breath Remedy (halitosis)

Get rid of the bacteria that cause bad breath with this effective remedy and enjoy fresh breath from day to day.

1tsp honey

¼ tsp cinnamon powder, ground

11/2 cup hot water

Instructions:

Mix the first two ingredients in the hot water and gargle 2 times daily.

Athlete's Foot Remedy

This common foot problem is caused by fungus growth and can be treated by a common remedy- Honey.

1. Apply a generous amount of honey on the affected area and rub thoroughly.

2. Wear an old pair of socks to cover feet before going to bed.

3. The following morning, wash feet off and dry.

4. Continue this treatment until the problem disappears.

Rosacea

Treat the blemishes and redness that accompanies Rosacea with honey

Raw honey

Little amount of distilled water

Instructions:

Mix together, apply to the face and leave for 3 hours or leave overnight.

Generally, redness and blemishes of Rosacea are difficult to treat, so be patient.

Burns

This treatment helps to prevent infections, redness and blisters. This is highly effective when the burn is immediately treated.

1. Apply a thin layer of honey on the burn and let it stay for 30 minutes. Wash off.

2. Apply to the affected area twice daily until the burn has healed.

3. Keep the area clean at all times to speed up the healing process.

Gum Disease

Clear up gum problems. Prevent them as well.

Instructions:

1. Brush your teeth. Massage honey on the gums for 5 minutes.

2. Do these 2 times a day. Alternatively, dilute honey with water and use as mouthwash

3. Additionally, you could add it to your toothpaste.

Eczema

No matter how stubborn or difficult your eczema, honey's several healing properties can handle it well.

Equal part honey

Equal part cinnamon

Instructions:

Mix and apply to affected area.

To prevent recurring eczema:

1 tsp honey

Juice of half lime or lemon

Instructions:

Add ingredients to 1cup water. Stir well and drink.

Eye Infection

Eye infection is caused by bacteria and thus can be treated with honey.

Equal parts honey

Equal parts distilled water

Instructions:

1. Mix and apply to eye with a cotton ball.

2. Leave on the eye for 30 minutes or apply as eye drops to the eye two times daily until the infection disappears.

Sinus Infection

Manuka honey destroys the germs that affect the sinus, throat and nose.

1 tsp Manuka honey

1/4 tsp baking soda

1/4 tsp sea salt, non-iodized

1 cup distilled water

Instructions:

1. Bring distilled water to a boil, add Manuka honey and stir. Next, add the baking soda and salt to it.

2. Let the mixture cool then pour it into a sterile container. Cover and refrigerate

3. using a sterile eye-dropper, apply the Manuka honey mixture by drawing it into the dropper, tilting your head back, and dispensing 8- 10 drops into the nostril.

4. Repeat as needed throughout the day.

5. For preventative purpose, take 1 teaspoon of Manuka oil orally every morning.

<u>Note</u>: Do not use Manuka honey if you suffer from bee sting allergies, tuberculosis, heart conditions or bee sting. If you are diabetic, see your doctor about the required dosage that is safe for you.

Indigestion

Honey promotes the growth of probiotics like Acidophillus and Bifidus which are essential for good digestion. It also helps to reduce stomach acid and quickly too.

1. Honey and lemon. Mix and drink.

2. To calm stomach, add honey to herbal tea.

Upset Stomach

With this remedy, your stomach troubles will be gone in no time.

1 tbsp honey

1 cup warm water

¼ tsp ground cinnamon

<u>Instructions:</u>

Add honey to warm water, mix well then add cinnamon to it.

Drink on an empty stomach

Ulcers (stomach and mouth)

Stomach ulcers are caused by Helicobacter pylori bacteria. Honey's antibacterial properties can help in treating this problem.

<u>Instructions</u>

1. Take 1 tbsp raw honey thrice daily with or without water.

2. It works for mouth ulcers as well.

Warts

1. Apply honey to wart then apply gauze on it.

2. Apply fresh honey daily until warts and scars disappear.

3. This can take up to 2 weeks.

Yeast Infection

1. Apply honey over affected area.

2. Let it stay for at 10 -15 minutes then rinse off.

3. Do this twice daily, in the morning and at night before bedtime.

HIDDEN WONDERS OF HONEY YOU NEVER THOUGHT OF

Honey Nail Strengthener

Get smooth, polished and stronger nails with this remedy

1 tbsp honey

¼ cup milk

2 egg yolks

Instructions:

1. In a small bowl, beat egg yolks and add milk and honey.

2. Place your nails inside this mixture for 10 to15 minutes.

3. Rinse your hands under cold running water and pat dry.

Get Rid Of Stress

The antioxidants in honey help to reduce stress levels.

1 tbsp honey

3 tbsp of warm water

Instructions

Mix ingredients, sip slowly and feel the stress disappear.

Sleeplessness/Insomnia

Having trouble sleeping? This remedy should help. It is extremely soothing and has a calming effect.

1 tsp honey

1 cup warm milk

Instructions

Combine and drink.

Honey For Insomnia: How It Works

Insomnia is dangerous for both children and adults because it comes with severe consequences such as mood swings, lack of concentration, obesity and severe health- related issues.

Nightly honey consumption leads to a little increase in blood sugar level and this leads to a controlled rise of insulin. When this happens, tryptophan, a sleep-promoting amino acid enters the brain. It gets converted to serotonin, a relaxing hormone. Now, once it gets dark, the serotonin converts to melatonin, which is widely used to cure sleeping disorders such as insomnia.

Another way that honey eliminates insomnia is by reducing stress hormones production at night. The body stores its energy source (glycogen) in the lever. Nevertheless, the liver may run out of glycogen at night.

When this happens, the brain triggers stress hormones like cortisol and adrenaline and the body will then be able to convert the protein muscle into glucose. The good thing is that honey is the best food for glycogen storage due to its ratio of fructose to glucose which is 1:1.

Asthma Relief

Asthma is caused by a variety of factors such as environmental conditions and allergies. However, honey offers tremendous relief.

1tsp honey

11/2tsp cinnamon

Instructions:

1. Mix well and consume. Alternatively, add mixture to 1 cup warm water.

2. Remedy is best taken before going to bed at night.

Memory Zest Blend

A mentally refreshing beverage for clarity and precision

Honey

1 part ginkgo

1 part rosemary leaves

1 part peppermint leaves and gotu kola

1 part ginger root

1 part red clover tops

Instructions:

1. Bring an entire tea pot or cup of water to a boil. Add the herbs.

2. Let the tea steep for 10-15 minutes, strain and add honey and drink.

Honey Lavender Lip Balm

1/2 tsp raw honey

1 tbsp shea butter

2 tbsp coconut oil

2 tbsp beeswax

1 tbsp sweet almond oil

5 drops Frankincense essential oil

15 drops Lavender essential oil

Equipment:

1 large rubber band

12 lip balm tubes

Instructions:

1. Take the lids out from the lip balm tubes and then secure them upright with the rubber band.

2. In a double boiler, gently melt the honey, coconut oil, beeswax and shea butter.

3. Take out from heat. Add the essential oils and sweet almond oil then stir.

4. Pour the melted oil immediately into the upright tubes.

5. Let the lip balm to set then close the containers.

Honey for Hangover

Honey calms the effects of the alcohol on the body and eliminates any cravings.

1. Upon waking, take 3-5teaspoons of honey. Depending on the severity of the hangover, keep on with this dose every 20 minutes.

2. At breakfast, take 4 more teaspoons.

Detoxification

Cleanse your system

21/2 tsp honey

1 lemon wedge

Instructions:

1. Add honey to I cup of boiling water. Stir well to dissolve.

2. Add the lemon wedge and drink.

Improve Your Immune System

Boost your immune system to be stronger against bacterial and viral attacks

2 tbsp honey

1 tsp cinnamon

Instructions:

Mix well and take.

Honey For Weight Loss

Take this drink when on a diet and when you crave something sweet.

1 tsp honey

1/2 tsp cinnamon powder

1 cup water

Instructions:

1. In a small saucepan, mix all three ingredients together.

2. Bring the mixture to a boil. Allow it to cool then refrigerate.

3. Take half of cup of this mixture 1 hour before breakfast. Take another half cup 1 hour before bedtime.

Tip: **How Honey Works For Weight Loss**

Honey is a natural energy-giving food. It works as a fat burner so it can be used as part of a recipe for weight loss. Sugar is highly processed so the nutrients benefits are minute, if at all in existence.

1 tsp sugar = 16 calories

1 tsp honey= 21 calories

Therefore, honey has a healthier glycemic index when compared to sugar. Thus when honey is consumed, it absorbs gradually into the body, providing you with a source of stabilized energy. You will not experience that energy crash or a sugar "high" afterwards.

Honey is also sweeter in taste compared to sugar. For this reason, less honey is needed. It is also more flavorful so add only a little to your food and drinks. Just a little bit of honey will satisfy you. This will keep you from cheating on your diet.

For individuals who are on a diet, exercising self control becomes easier to achieve. Simply take a little bit of honey and your 'sweet tooth' will be effortlessly satisfied. Honey helps with the low energy levels experienced by most people on a diet. With honey consumption, your energy level is stabilized all through the day.

Honey For Lower Cholesterol

Bad cholesterol (LDL) levels can now be lowered with honey as honey contains lots of antioxidants which stops plague from accumulating on blood vessel walls.

1tsp honey

1 cup warm water

Instructions:

Mix well and drink daily

How Honey Lowers Cholesterol In The Body

Cholesterol is essential to several human functions. For instance, it helps to produce many hormones that are used in several cell membranes. In spite of its significance, high cholesterol is risky to the heart and likely to cause heart attack.

The wonders of honey in lowering cholesterol in the body

Honey contains nutrients that fight the cholesterol in the body. Calcium, sodium, potassium and vitamin B complex are a few of these nutrients. Honey also contains antioxidants that help in increasing the level of blood within the body especially when it is taken daily.

It can also help to clean the blood vessels consequently lowering the chances of high blood pressure in body. This is definitely better than any health enhancement supplements available.

Honey For Diabetes Solution

Honey does not raise blood sugar levels in the same way table sugar does. Therefore, diabetics are usually advised to eat foods that contain plenty of vitamins C, E, B1, B12, B6 as well as Biotin.

All these nutrients can be found in any good quality honey.

Honey For Exercise

Exercise is important to keep fit and for weight loss. When you eat honey, you get the needed energy. Research has shown that athletes who eat some honey after their performance recover faster. Reducing heart attack incidences becomes easier as well.

So get into the habit of taking a little honey when going to the gym or going for a walk. You will be able to endure vigorous exercises

Instructions:

1. 1 tsp of raw honey added to your water bottle is all that you need.

2. You will feel real good after the workout.

FORMS OF HONEY

Freezing Honey

Freezing honey is the best way to store it. Overtime, honey ages and loses its color and flavor. Honey should never be refrigerated as it will change flavor and granulate and you may eventually have to throw it away.

Instructions

1. Divide the honey into small amounts as it is pointless to freeze the entire bottle then thawing it all when needed.

2. Freeze honey in a sealed glass container. (Plastic container may affect the flavor of the honey).

3. Place a label with the freezing date of the honey neatly pasted on it. This will help you to know the container of honey to use first.

4. Don't remove the honey from the freezer until you are ready to use it. Give the honey plenty of time to thaw.

Preventing Crystallization Of Honey

Crystallization is the process of solidifying honey. Honey that is kept in the freezer will not solidify as a result of its low moisture content. Glucose content in honey is less soluble than fructose so it will crystallize when it is separated from the water.

To dissolve the crystals, the honey can be placed in the microwave but it is better to prevent crystallization completely.

Freezing honey prevents crystallization, although it may have to be thawed before it can be poured easily.

Things You'll Need

Honey

Plastic wrap

Ice cube tray

Instructions

1. Pour the honey into an ice cube tray. (A larger container should be used if you are using large amounts of honey at the same time).

2. Use the plastic wrap to wrap the ice cube tray or container and then place in the freezer. The honey will become very thick but will not freeze. (The plastic wrap stops other freezer odors from entering into the honey. Also, if the tray tips, the freezer will remain clean).

3. Remove the number of cubes that is needed, leave them to thaw on your counter or place them straight into your recipe. Each cube holds about 1 tablespoon.

4. An entire honey container can also be frozen; defrost for 30-40 minutes before using.

Hardening Honey

Honey eventually hardens or crystallizes naturally due to small particles of sugar, wax, crumbs or pollen that enable the honey crystals to form.

Crystallization doesn't mean that the honey has gone bad. As a matter of fact, honey stored in a cool environment when opened remains fit for human consumption for at least 10 years. Unopened honey is indefinitely edible.

Some people enjoy crystallized or hardened honey because the water content evaporates and this intensifies the sweetness. However, if you cannot wait for the honey to crystallize naturally, cook it to a toffee-like consistency then make lozenges.

Things You'll Need

1/2 cup honey

2 cups sugar

1 tbsp vinegar

1/4 cup water

Double boiler

Instructions

1. Pour water in the bottom of a double boiler then bring to a boil. Lower heat

2. Add water, honey, vinegar and sugar in the second pan and place it into the boiling water. (The sugar allows the honey to crystallize when the solution cools).

3. Bring second pan to a boil. Reduce to a simmer. Constantly stir so it doesn't stick.

4. Once the solution gets to about 300 degrees F, carry out a hard-crack test. Fill a glass cup with cool water. Add a spoonful of the honey into the water to cool. The honey should immediately snap when you remove it after cooling,

5. If it bends or rolls into a ball before breaking, keep heating and do the test again after 1- 2 minutes.

6. Take out the pan of honey from the double boiler. Divide the thickened honey before it cools.

PART III: Baking Soda

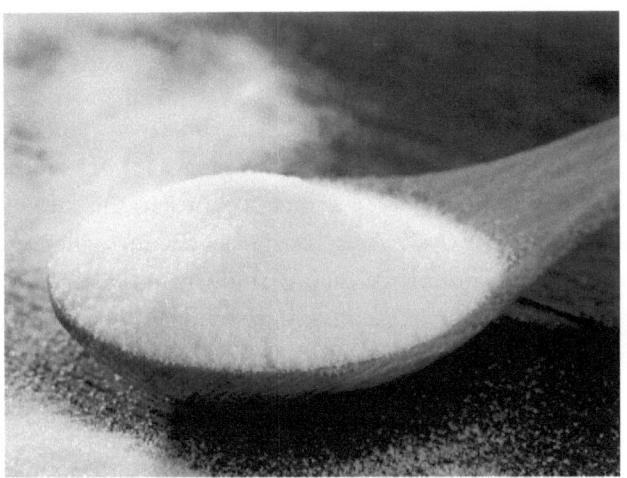

An Insight Into The Wonders Of Baking Soda

Baking soda is a white powder with an alkaline taste. Also known as sodium bicarbonate, bicarbonate of soda and bicarb, it is readily available as it is found naturally dissolved in mineral springs all over the world. Baking soda is incredibly versatile and amazingly cheap particularly when purchased in bulk. Originally meant for cooking, it has proven to be highly useful in various ways, including cleaning and medical purposes.

When used in cooking, baking soda acts as a leavening agent that causes baked goods to rise. Once it is added to the batter, it reacts with an acidic ingredient in the recipe such as honey, lemon juice, milk or brown sugar. This reaction creates carbon dioxide that expands the dough and as it bakes, it rises. It is used in baking breads, cakes and cookies.

As a cleaning agent, it is safe and contains no toxic substances that could be detrimental to health - both of humans and pets. While a lot of commercial household cleaners are petroleum-based and contributes to the further depletion of our natural resources, baking soda is environmentally friendly and the safest choice to conventional cleaning products in the market. As a matter of fact, it is incomparable to the highly scented commercial products that are usually filled with unpronounceable chemical ingredients that are dangerous to health.

Baking Soda is the perfect all-purpose cleaner for the home. It dissolves dirt in water, cuts grease and lifts oils and discoloration with ease. It also lifts up buildup on scalps from conditioners, hairsprays, and other products. It is a food-safe cleaner that can safely be used to clean every surface in the home. With a little water added to it, it can be made into a paste or used dry. It does a great job of scouring pots, pans, ovens, stovetops among others.

As a deodorizing agent, it neutralizes all kinds of odors. Causative agents of the unpleasant odors such as strong acids from spoiled milk or strong bases from spoilt fish are effectively neutralized. Baking soda brings the acidic and basic odor molecules into an odor-free and neutral state, thus acting as a deodorizer. Baking soda also deodorizes when dissolved in water and can be used as a mouthwash to deodorize bad breathe or on plastic food containers to deodorize absorbed pickle smells.

Baking soda acts as a buffer. It helps to maintain a stable acid-alkali balance or pH (power of hydrogen) balance. This keeps the substance neither too alkaline nor too acidic. Water is neutral with a pH of 7, acids have a pH that is less than 7 while alkaline solutions have a pH that is higher than 7. When baking soda comes in contact with an acidic or alkaline substance, it naturally neutralizes that pH.

Baking soda can cause acid solutions to become more basic and basic solutions to become more acid. Thus, it helps in balancing the acid in our body by neutralizing the stomach acid to relieve us of acid indigestion, sour stomach and heartburn. It also works the same way on irritated skin by soothing inflammation and relieving itches and pain.

It is advisable to use a brand of baking soda that is aluminum- free. This is not difficult to find as most of them are. However, there are still quite a few that may be contaminated with aluminum so it is better to be 100 percent sure and safe. Baking soda is a wonder and a quick solution to numerous household issues.

Why Use Baking Soda

Below are a few reasons you should use baking soda instead of the conventional cleaning products. Once you go through these information, you will definetely do away with chemical household cleaners once and for all!

It Is Toxic-Free

Nowadays, many store-bought cleaning products contain a lot of harmful toxins. It is dangerous to inhale or use these products. Harmful chemicals that may be contained in them include ammonia, perchloroethylene, chlorine and phthalates. Excessive use of these chemicals may cause cancer and lung damage.

Other ways chemicals in conventional cleaners may endanger human health include:

Damaging the kidney and liver

- Causing chemical burns in the sinuses and esophagus.
- Damaging organs from skin exposure.
- Damaging the skin from prolonged exposure.
- Causing throat irritation.
- Swelling of the mouth and throat.
- Headaches and dizziness

It is Safe For Kids

Isn't it a great relief that you no longer need to be unduly worried about your kids stumbling on chemical cleaners or wondering whether you have kept the cabinets unlocked or left any chemicals out of the reach of an inquisitive child?

While you still need to lock up your non- toxic cleaning products in cabinets with child-proof locks, you are now less likely to worry about causing your children major health damage even if they come in contact with them.

Now not only are you worry-free but your kids can also follow you around, watch and even offer to help while you clean. It is also a great opportunity for you to teach them how to scrub the bathroom counters as they watch and imitate your move with a sponge.

... And Pets Too

Pets are at risk of inhaling and even directly ingesting toxic cleaning products. With their noses so close to the ground, they will sniff, lick and lay in spilled toxic cleaners. In the long run, these animals will suffer numerous health problems. You ought to protect these animals by switching to natural cleaners and keep them perpetually healthy.

Breathe Clean Air

Store-bought household cleaners being full of toxic chemicals pollute the air. After all, don't most of them come with warning labels about not directly breathing in the fumes? Sadly however, it is inhaled indirectly because they tend to linger in the air for a while. Furthermore, research has proven that the air quality inside a lot of homes can be two times to five times more contaminated than the air outside our homes. And this is caused by the household cleaners we use from day to day.

...And Drink Clean Water

Traditional cleaners seep into our water. The thing is, once you use them to clean, the volatile chemicals they contain get into the greater water cycle. While water treatment plants help to purify most of this water, it is difficult for them to effectively treat a large volume of these chemicals. Eventually, they find their way back to the water you use in your home. So you see, you may be unknowingly contributing to a poisoned water supply. This is another reason you should go green so you do not add toxins and poisons back into the environment that produces the water.

Save Money- It's Good For Your Pocket

Most natural cleaning recipes are inexpensive. Baking soda, for instance is amazingly cheap it's almost a steal! They are even cheaper when bought in bulk. When compared to their synthetic counterparts, you get to save some good money at the end of every month. They are easy to make as well, they will not take you much time, put one or two ingredients together and viola, you are good to go. The ingredients are readily available in grocery stores.

Get The Job Done- Naturally

Natural cleaners work! They have been tested and proven several times to be just as effective as synthetic cleaning products. It makes a lot of sense to switch as it still gets the job done.

Kitchen Cleaning With Baking Soda

Food Safe/Surface Safe kitchen

Why use harsh chemicals on your sinks, dish strainers and counters when dinner will still be made on those same surfaces?! Simply sprinkle Baking Soda on a damp cloth, wipe clean, rinse thoroughly and dry.

You can also use this on cutting boards to eliminate onion smells and odors from previous cooking, backsplashes, plastic containers, microwaves, range hoods, oven tops and more!

By using this simple cleaning method, your kitchen will be clean and fresh.

Cleaning Coffee and Tea Pots

Remove coffee and tea stains and get rid of bitter off-tastes by combining these 2 ingredients:

1/4 cup Baking Soda

1 quart warm water

For stubborn stains, add a little detergent in the solution soak overnight.

Remove unsightly stains from mugs and cups by scrubbing with sponge sprinkled with baking soda.

Deodorizing Dishwashers

Not ready to wash the dishes yet?

Sprinkle some Baking Soda in the bottom of the dishwasher or directly on the dishes to absorb the odors from the dishes. The baking soda does 2 things:

1. Deodorizes before the dishwasher is run and

2. Cleaning in the first wash cycle.

Easier Dish Washing

Bolster your liquid's detergent's cleaning power. Add 2 tablespoons of baking soda to the dish water or sink along with the detergent. This will help to cut food and grease on pots, pans and dishes.

Control dishwasher odors by simply sprinkling a little baking soda on the bottom of the dishwasher between loads.

Drains and Garbage Disposals

Deodorize drains and disposal by pouring Baking Soda down your drain while running warm tap water. The Baking Soda works by neutralizing acid and basic odors so you could have a fresh drain.

For your slow drains, pour about 1 cup soda down the drain, pour about 1/2 cup of salt and then pour boiling water over it. Drain should now run well with no nasty smell.

Sprinkle Baking Soda in garbage cans to minimize the smell. Sprinkle between layers of garbage as they accumulate.

You should also wash and deodorize garbage cans occasionally by making a solution of 1 cup of Baking Soda for every 1 gallon of water.

Fruit And Vegetable Scrub

Clean off residue and dirt on fresh fruit and vegetables. Sprinkle baking soda on a damp sponge, scrub and rinse. It's safe! Enjoy your fruits and veggies.

Pots & Pans Care

Thanks to Baking Soda, no more heavy scrubbing of pots and pans! Simply combine baking soda, hot water and dish detergent and pour on pots and pans. Let it sit for 10 minutes and then wash.

Alternatively, sprinkle baking soda on roasting pans and crusted casseroles and let sit for five minutes. Scrub and rinse gently.

Soften burnt-on food by sprinkling a generous amount of baking soda over pots and pans' surfaces. Add hot water and leave to soak for 10 minutes. Add baking soda to damp sponge and scrub.

Microwave Cleaning

Clean and deodorize your microwave. Add 4 tablespoons of Baking Soda to 1 quart water. Use this solution and then rinse with clear water.

Refrigerators

Baking soda works for exterior and interior cleaning of your refrigerator.

Dissolve 2 tablespoons of baking soda in 1 quart warm water. Wipe all surfaces.

For stubborn areas, use baking soda and water paste to clean.

Deodorize your refrigerator: open a box of baking soda and place inside. Replace after three months.

Kitchen Sink& Sponges

Clean your kitchen sink by sprinkling baking soda into it and add a little vinegar. Once it starts to bubble, scrub the sink with a brush and rinse.

Soak stale-smelling sponges in a strong baking Soda solution to keep them fresh.

Deodorizing Containers

Baking soda can keep your plastic food containers and thermos smelling fresh.

Sprinkle baking soda on damp sponge and wash items or add 2 tbsp baking soda to container, fill it with hot water, cover and shake well.

For strong odors, prepare a solution of 4 tbsp Baking Soda and 1 quart of warm water. Soak items in it. You will be amazed at the outcome!

Silverware Shiner/ Homemade Ash Metal Polish

Add equal parts baking soda and equal parts warm water together to make paste. Using a sponge, apply to silver. Rub, rinse, and buff dry.

To make a metal ash polish, combine 4 tablespoons baking soda and 2 cups wood ashes from a woodstove or fireplace. Add just enough water to make a paste. Dampen a sponge and use it to rub the mixture onto stainless steel, chrome, gold or silver plating. Rinse and dry.

Extinguishing Minor Fires

Use Baking soda to smother small flames in the kitchen. It works because heated baking soda gives off carbon dioxide, which helps to smother grease and electrical fires.

For small cooking fires from ovens, burners, fry-pans, broilers and grills, turn off electricity or gas (if you can do so safely). Stand back and toss handfuls of baking Soda at the base of the flame to put the fire out.

For small electrical fires from heaters, outlets and small appliances, unplug appliances if you can do so safely. Then stand back and toss handfuls of baking Soda at the base of the flame to put the fire out.

In both instances, call the fire department afterwards to ensure the fire is out. To avoid re- ignition, do not try to move the item until completely cooled. Never use water on electrical fires because it could lead to electrocution or shock. Never use Baking Soda in deep fat fryers so it does not splatter.

Bathroom Cleaning With Baking Soda

Bathroom Floor Cleaner

Baking Soda dissolves the grime and dirt from a bathroom tile or no-wax floor easily and quickly.

Add 1/2 cup Baking Soda to a bucket of warm water, mixing well.

Mop floor or tile and rinse clean. Let your floor sparkle.

Shiny Tiles & Sinks

Sprinkle a little Baking Soda on a damp sponge. Scrub sink, tile and tub as usual. Rinse well and wipe dry.

Homemade Bathroom Scrub

Mix ¼ cup of baking soda and 1 tablespoon of liquid detergent together. Add a little vinegar to make it thick and creamy. Use as needed.

Toothbrush Soak

Add ¼ cup baking soda to ¼ cup water, mixing thoroughly. Soak toothbrushes in mixture and let them stand overnight for a good cleaning.

Shower Curtains & Toilet bowl

To deodorize and clean your shower curtain, sprinkle Baking Soda on a damp brush. Scrub shower curtain, rinse clean and hang it up to dry.

To clean the toilet bowl, toss 1/2 cup of baking soda into it and scour with toilet brush.

Grout & Tile Stains Remover

Add 3 parts baking soda to 1part water to make paste. Apply to grout with toothbrush or with damp sponge.

Hard Bathwater Softener

Add 1/2 cup of baking soda to your bath water and enjoy a relaxing and deodorizing soak

Septic Care

Help your Septic System flow freely by treat the septic tank with baking soda.

Flush 1 cup of Baking Soda down the toilet every week to help maintain a good pH in your septic tank.

Laundry With Baking Soda

Your laundry room can do with baking soda. Here are ways to go about it:

Freshen Laundry Hampers

Keep the clothes hamper fresh until ready to wash by sprinkling a generous amount of baking soda between clothes layers. This also softens the clothes at wash time.

During washing, add 1/2 cup Baking Soda with your favorite detergent to freshen laundry and help liquid detergents work harder!

Stubborn Smell Remover

Remove stubborn and sour smells from clothes such as perspiration odors, musty smells from storage and sour towels used in the summer by adding 1/2 cup of Baking Soda to the rinse cycle. Your clothes will emerge clean and smelling fresh.

Alternatively, you can treat smelly clothes before wash time by soaking them for at least an hour in a solution of 1/2 cup baking soda and 1 gallon of warm water.

Chlorine Bleach Booster

Baking Soda will help your liquid chlorine bleach to work harder. Your whites will be whiter and fresher. Just add 1/2 cup Baking Soda to your usual amount of liquid bleach. For front loaders, add 1/4 cup.

Freshen Closets

Place a box of baking soda on the closet shelf to keep clothes smelling fresh.

Excellent Baby Laundry

Spits-up occur often. When it does, rub baking soda over bibs to cut odors and make laundry easier. To freshen cloth diapers, soak in a solution of 1/2 cup baking soda and 2 quarts of water. To clean and deodorize diaper pail, combine baking soda and water then use it to wipe the inside and outside of the pail.

Homemade Fabric Softener

Combine 1 cup baking soda, 6 cups distilled white vinegar and 8 cups water. This makes about a gallon and you can use 1 cup per regular load of laundry in the last rinse cycle.

Pets, Toys And Pests

Porcupine Quill Remover
Add 2 teaspoons baking soda to 1 cup vinegar and apply to quill area.

After 10 minutes, reapply and wait again for 10 minutes. Quills should come from your pets easily.

Fido Dry-Cleaner
Baking soda is non-toxic and therefore safe to use around dogs. Rub a handful of baking soda into dog's fur and then comb it out. Dog will be clean and deodorized even without a bath. To brush your pets' teeth, add baking soda to toothbrush and use.

Toys And Dishes Cleaner
Soak your pet's dishes and toys in a solution of 3 tbsp baking soda and1 quart warm water. Keep pests away from your Fido's food bowls by surrounding bowl with baking soda.

Pet Bedding & Cages
Sprinkle baking soda over dry surface. Let it sit for 15 minutes, then vacuum. To clean small animal cage, sprinkle baking soda on damp sponge and wipe surfaces. Rinse and dry.

Keep Ants At Bay
Combine equal parts of baking soda and water. Sprinkle mixture where there are ants.

Roaches And Silverfish Killer

Mix equal parts baking soda and sugar together. Place in an infected area. Bugs like sugar and will be drawn to them and end up eating too much baking soda which will kill them.

Fresh Kitty Litter

Spread baking soda on the bottom of kitty box. Cover with litter to maximize smells. Alternatively, make a litter by adding a small box of baking soda to 3 inches of sandy clay, mixing thoroughly.

Toys &Stuffed Animal Freshener

Keep cuddly stuffed animals fresh by sprinkling baking soda on them and leaving for 15 minutes. Simply brush off afterwards.

Clean other toys by using 1/4 cup baking soda and 1 quart warm water. Submerge these toys in this mixture and then rinse with clear water. You can also dampen a cloth with this mixture and wipe toys.

Hygiene And Beauty Uses With Baking Soda

Mouthwash/Bad Breath Killer

Make a mouthwash with baking soda by adding 1 teaspoon of it to 1/2 glass of water. Swish through teeth and rinse. For those who suffer from bad breath, this solution is highly effective as baking soda does more just covering up the smell cause by bacteria but neutralizes it.

If you prefer a slightly more effective mouthwash that can kill bacteria and prevent gum disease and infection, add a pinch of salt to the solution. This is because salt (sodium) is disinfectant and kills off germs.

Homemade Toothpaste

Baking Soda is a mild dentifrice that helps to keep teeth white and clean.

To brush your teeth the natural way, add a little baking soda on a wet toothbrush and brush as usual. This will clean teeth and neutralize bacterial waste.

Dentures/ Retainers Freshener

Soak dentures, retainers, mouthpieces and other oral appliance in 2 teaspoons of Baking Soda and a small bowl of warm water. The Baking Soda works by loosening food particles and neutralizing odors to keep dentures or retainers fresh.

Refreshing Bath Additive

Have a refreshing bath. Add 1/2 cup of Baking Soda to your tub of water. The Baking Soda works by neutralizing acids on the skin and washing away oil and perspiration. Relax, enjoy your bath and emerge with skin that feels silky soft.

De-product Hair

When your favorite shampoo or conditioner no longer works on your hair, the likely cause is product build-up on your hair. Say goodbye to build-ups from mousses, sprays and conditioners with the help of baking soda.

Simply add1 teaspoon of Baking Soda to your regular shampoo bottle and wash hair. This will give you a natural clean hair and prevent product build ups well.

Alternatively, after shampooing hair, dissolve teaspoon baking soda in 1 cup of water or apple cider vinegar. Pour this mixture over your hair and rinse off with fresh, clean water.

Dry shampoo

To remove excess oils in your hair, dust hair with dry baking soda. This helps when you do not feel like shampooing. Use as a dry shampoo.

Hand Cleanser

Neutralize odors on hands and scour away ground-in dirt with a paste of 3 parts Baking soda added to 1 part water. Alternately use 3 parts Baking Soda added to 1 part liquid hand soap. Scrub and then rinse clean.

Nails Cleanser

Yellowing, stained nails are unsightly and can make your hands look older. Make a paste of equal parts baking soda and hydrogen peroxide. Afterwards, use a nail scrub brush to scrub on top of your nails and under it. Leave to sit for about 5 minutes and then rinse off. However, if your nails are persistently yellow, consult a doctor as this could be a sign of a fungal infection.

All- Natural Facial Scrub

Baking Soda can be used as an invigorating and gentle, facial scrub. Simply make a baking soda paste of 3 parts to 1 part water. Wash face with soap and water and then apply in a gentle circular motion. Rinse clean.

Soothing Foot Soak

Are your feet tired? Soak them for 10 minutes in a solution of 4 tbsp baking soda and 1 qt. warm water. It also provides relief from itchiness caused by athlete's foot and helps to soften calluses.

Natural Deodorant

Searching for a natural alternative to sticks and sprays? A pinch baking soda sprinkled under your arms will do. Alternatively, you may make a paste by mixing with water and if you cannot make it stick, add a little cornstarch to it.

To deodorize your shoes, simple sprinkle some baking soda in them. Baking soda also helps to minimize razor burns before and after shaving. Just add 1 tablespoon baking soda to 1 cup of water and apply to face.

Grooming Accessories Cleaner

Soak combs, brushes, cosmetic sponges, curlers and applicators overnight in a solution of 4 tablespoons baking soda and 1 quart of water. Rinse and leave to dry. This helps to clean hair product residue and natural oil build-up from such accessories like combs and brushes.

Silver Jewelry Polisher

Does your silver jewelry look old and tarnished? Try this recipe.

Pour very hot water into a small bowl and dip your jewelry in it. Now add 1 tablespoon of baking soda and 1 sheet of aluminum foil in the water. By doing this, the tarnish from your jewelry is transferred to the aluminum. Using a wooden device, move the pieces around, ensuring that the jewelry touches the aluminum. After a few minutes, rinse jewelry and polish with a soft cloth. Do not use this on organic material like pearls or jewelry with gemstones to avoid damage.

Personal Health Care With Baking Soda

Soothe minor burns and rashes

Make a paste by combining 3parts baking soda, 1 part witch hazel or water and apply. Recipe can be used for poison ivy itch as well.

Baking soda also helps to clear acne. Simply make a paste and spread it over your face. It works like magic!

Antacid Drug

Dissolve 1/2 teaspoon of baking soda in 1/2 glass of water. Drink slowly.

Insect Bite Care

Make a Baking Soda paste and ease the pain and itching cause by an insect bite.

1. Remove the stinger.

2. Combine 3 parts Baking Soda to 1 part water and apply to the area affected.

3. Leave to dry, wash off and repeat if necessary.

Soothe Irritated Skin

Baking Soda helps to soothe the sting of minor burns, sunburn and windburn.

Make a baking soda solution of 4 tablespoons in 1 quart of water. Immerse a washcloth in the solution and apply to the affected area.

Alternatively, make a paste with 3 parts Baking Soda and 1 part water and then apply to the area.

Soothing Skin Bath

Add 1/2 cup Baking Soda to a bath of water. Enjoy your bath and be relieved of the itchy skin of poison ivy or prickly heat.

For localized rashes and irritations, make a paste using 3 parts Baking Soda and 1 part water.

Treat diaper rash by putting 2 tablespoons of bathing soda in your baby's bathwater.

Sore Throat Eliminator

Ease your sore throat by making a solution of baking soda and water and gargling every 4 hours. This works because baking soda eliminates the acids causing the pain.

Stuffy Nose

Add 1teaspoon of baking soda to your vaporizer. This will unblock your stuffy nose fast!

Neutralize Gassy Beans

Prevent gassy issue and aid digestion. Soak your beans as usual then sprinkle 1teaspoon of baking soda in the water.

Around The Home With Baking Soda

Scuff Marks Remover/ Safer Front Steps

Remove scuff marks on your no-wax floor. Sprinkle Baking Soda on damp sponge, rub clean and then rinse. Baking Soda removes scuff marks without scratching the floor!

Skid-proof front steps by sprinkling baking soda liberally on icy steps and walkways.

Musty Books Deodorizer

Dry the books out then sprinkle a little baking soda between pages. Let it stay for 5 to 7 days then brush out.

Cleaner Walls & Carpets

Crayon marks from walls can be gently removed with baking soda. Rub with a damp sponge or cloth sprinkled with baking soda.

Deodorize your carpets. Sprinkle a lot of baking soda on carpets then leave for 15 minutes. Go ahead and vacuum.

Deodorize Smoke-Filled Room

Eliminate the haze and odor from your room by adding 1quart of warm water and 4tablespoons baking soda to a plant mister. Spray into the smoky air.

Fresher& Longer Lasting Flowers

Your cut flowers can be fresher and made to last longer with baking soda. Just add 1teaspoon of it to the water in the vase and that's it.

Make An Inexpensive Plaster

To make a plaster, make a paste by combining white glue and baking soda. Apply to cracks with a finger.

Shoes, Rubber Gloves & Chairs

To polish white baby shoes, sprinkle baking soda on them and rub with a damp sponge. Rinse shoes and buff.

Sweeten smelly sneakers by just sprinkling a little baking soda inside. Shake out before wearing.

If you are finding it hard to slip into your rubbers gloves after trying repeatedly, simply rub some baking soda into the fingers then you will be able to slip them on easily.

Clean your baby's high chair by using a solution of 4 tablespoons of baking soda in 1 quart of warm water. For really stained or very dirty ones, scrub directly with baking soda on a damp sponge.

Air Freshener

Mix baking soda with any perfumed bath salts that you choose. Transfer the mixture into small sachet bags and place indoors. The air will be freshened.

Cars And Garages

Batteries Cleaner

Baking Soda is a mild alkali. Therefore, it can help to neutralize battery acid corrosion on cars. Begin by disconnecting the battery terminals then add 3parts Baking Soda and 1 part water together to form a paste.

Dampen a cloth and use to scrub corroded battery terminal. Re-connect the terminals once done then coat with petroleum jelly so corrosion does not occur again. A word of caution: batteries contain strong acid so be careful when working around them.

Cleaner Cars

Clean your car lights, windows, chrome, vinyl seats, tires and floor mats with baking soda.

Add Baking Soda to 1 quart warm water and apply this solution with a soft cloth or sponge to remove tree sap, road grime, tar and bugs.

For stubborn stains, sprinkle baking Soda onto a damp sponge and use. Rinse and then dry with a soft towel. The result is a clean and toxic-free car with streak-free windshield, freshened floor mats and brightened headlights.

Oil and Grease Stains Remover

Clean up grease spills and light-duty oil in your driveway or garage floor. Just sprinkle Baking soda directly on the spot and use a wet brush to scrub.

Cars Deodorizers

Eliminate odors from upholstery and carpets. Sprinkle baking Soda directly on them. Wait for at least 15 minutes and then vacuum.

Deodorize Car Ashtrays

To eliminate stale tobacco odors, just pour 1/2 inch of Baking Soda in the ashtray. It will also help in extinguishing cigarettes and cigars. Replace Baking Soda weekly and empty ashtrays regularly.

RV Water Tanks Deodorizer

Protect your RV against rancid taste and sweeten it. Fill reservoir with 1 cup of baking soda dissolved in 1 gallon of warm water. Drain and flush then fill tank with plain water. Drain again and fill again with plain water. This works because the baking soda eliminates stale odors as well as the mineral buildup that leads to it.

Baking Soda For Outdoor Use

Cleaning Grills

Clean up grill for the next barbecue. Sprinkle a little dry baking soda on a damp brush, scrub gently and rinse clean. Baking Soda won't scratch shiny surfaces and it cleans exterior surfaces such as trays and knobs very well.

Pool Care

Maintain a balanced swimming pool pH. The right pH protects the walls of your pools, its metal fittings and makes swimming in the water delightful instead of an itchy and unpleasant experience. A pH of 7.4 to 7.8 is the appropriate range for a swimming pool. However, if the pH of your pool registers as low after testing it, you can use baking soda to slightly raise your pH but do not to add too much baking soda because it is harder to lower total alkalinity than it is to raise it.

Baking soda's main task is to raise the total alkalinity of a pool. If the pH in your pool keeps dropping even after trying to raise it, test your total alkalinity. Total alkalinity should be between 80 ppm to 150 ppm. With low total alkalinity, the pH will fluctuates at random. If your test indicates a low total alkalinity, add 1.4 lbs of baking soda per 10,000 gallons of water in your swimming pool. This should increase the total alkalinity by at least10 ppm. Allow the water circulate for 1- 2 hours before testing again.

Cleaner Pool Tools

Clean plastic and vinyl pool toys and eliminates any mildew-like odors. Make a solution of 1/4 cup Baking Soda and1 quart warm water. Wipe down and rinse. For very dirty toys, dampen a sponge, sprinkle some baking Soda on it, scrub item and rinse.

Non-Toxic Homemade Fungicide

Add 4 teaspoons baking soda to 1 gallon of water. Spray on vines and grapes at the appearance of the first fruits. Spray once in a week for 2 months, and after each rain. It can also be sprayed on rosebushes to fight black spot fungus.

Rejuvenate The Greenery

Add 1 teaspoon of baking soda, 1 teaspoon of Epsom salt, 1/2 teaspoon of clear ammonia together in a gallon of water. For each rosebush-size shrub, use about1 quart of this solution and watch it regain its luster after a while.

Your beloved veggies are susceptible to consumption by rabbits. To prevent this from happening, spread baking soda around your flowerbeds.

You can also sweeten your tomatoes by sprinkling some baking soda around your tomato plants.

Power Cleaner

Spruce up your fishing gear by making baking soda solution and then using it to clean rods, hooks, lines and buckets. There's no need to worry as baking soda will not pollute rivers and lakes. Cleanse your hands from gardening grime by rubbing baking soda on wet hands and rinsing afterwards.

Clean Lawn Furniture

Add 1/4 cup of Baking Soda to 1 quart of warm water. Use this solution to clean and deodorize patio and pool furniture. Rinse clean.

For tougher stains, sprinkle the baking Soda directly on a damp cloth or sponge, scrub and rinse.

The End